ESSENTIAL GUIDE TO PITYRIASIS ROSEA

Understanding, Managing, and Treating the Condition

DR. CASEY LOREN

DISCLAIMER

This book's content is only meant to be used for general informative purposes. Although the author has taken great care to ensure the content is accurate and thorough, no warranties or assurances on the information's accuracy, correctness, or reliability are provided. It is recommended that readers employ their own judgment and discretion when applying any material found in this book to their particular situation.

The information in this book is not intended to replace professional advice, nor is the author an expert in any of the subjects covered. It is recommended that readers consult with experienced professionals regarding any particular issues or concerns.

Any name that may be mentioned or referred in this book does not imply endorsement, recommendation, or relationship on the part of the author with any person, entity, good, website, or association. These references are made only for informational purposes and are not meant to be taken as recommendations or endorsements.

The information contained in this book may cause readers to suffer loss or damage, for which the author disclaims all obligation and accountability. The only people accountable for the decisions and actions taken by readers using the information presented are themselves.

Any names, characters, companies, locations, activities, occasions, and incidents referenced in this book are either made up or the result of the author's imagination. Any likeness to real people, living or dead, or to real things is entirely coincidental.

This book's content may change at any time, without prior notice, according to the author. The onus is on the reader to verify whether there have been any updates or revisions.

The reader accepts the conditions of this disclaimer by reading this book. Please do not read this book or use its contents if you do not agree to these terms.

Table of Contents

CHAPTER 1..14

PITYRIASIS ROSEA: A BRIEF OVERVIEW 14

Preface and Definition 14

The Past and Its Impact 14

Research on the Causes and Rates of Pityriasis Rosea 15

Causes and Potential Hazards 15

Its Symptoms and Clinical Presentation 16

Possible Diagnosis...16

Techniques for Diagnosis 17

Concerns and Future Outlook.......................17

Approaches to Treatment 18

Education and Support for Patients 18

CHAPTER 2..20

SKIN PHYSIOLOGY AND ANATOMY 20

Skin Structure..20

The Skin and Its Functions: 21

The Language of Dermatology:.....................21

Taking Care of Your Skin and Immune System:..22

How Hormones Affect Skin Disorders:........22

Skin Disorders and Heredity:.....................23

Matters Influencing the Skin from the Environment:..24

Skin Alterations as a Result of Ageing: 24

How to Take Care of Your Skin: 25

How Your Diet Affects Your Skin's Condition: 26

CHAPTER 3..28

HOW PITYRIASIS ROSEA DEVELOPS 28

How Pityriasis Rosea Develops 28

The Immunological Processes At Work.......28

Things That Can Set Off a Virus and How It Can Spread..29

Cytokines and T Cells: Their Function.........29

Determinants of Autoimmune Diseases 30

The Role of Heredity 30

Impacts on the Environment 30

Factors related to hormones 31

Changes in Skin Lesions Caused by Pathology

....31

Reactions Causing Inflammation 31

CHAPTER 4..34

FACTORS AND VARIANTS IN CLINICAL

PRACTICE 34

Pityriasis rosea in its traditional form: 34

Unusual and Atypical Variants:....................34

Progression and Clinical Stages....................35

Skin Lesion Morphology................................36

Patterns of Distribution:...............................36

Signs & Symptoms, Including Itching: 36

Differences in Display Based on Gender and

Age:...37

Effects on People's Standard of Living:........37

Effects on the Mind and Emotions: 38

Consequences in the Long Run:....................38

CHAPTER 5 40

ASSESSMENT FOR DIAGNOSIS 40

Evaluating the Clinical 40

Evaluation of Skin Conditions 41

Options for Contemplating a Different Diagnosis..42

Results from Histopathology......................44

The lack of major systemic symptoms 46

A Critical Aspect of Prompt Identification ...47

CHAPTER 6 50

METHODS FOR CONTROL AND REHABILITATION 50

A Primer on Management Theory and Practice 50

Counseling and Education for Patients 51

Pharmaceutical Approaches 51

Treatments Applied Topically 52

Systemic therapies 52

Non-Conventional and Allied Medical Practices 53

Managing Itching..53

Complication Prevention...............................54

Care Maintenance 55

Factors that Predict Outcome.......................55

CHAPTER 7 58

PSYCHOSOCIAL EFFECTS AND METHODS OF COPING 58

How Pityriasis Rosea Affects the Mind:.......58

Effects on Confidence and Perception of One's Body: 58

Methods for Coping and Resources for Help: 59

Things to Think About for Your Mental Health: 59

Psychotherapy and Counselling:..................60

Family and social support play an important role:..61

Programmes for Raising Awareness and Education: 61

Promoting Patients' Legal Rights:................62

Confronting Misconceptions and Stigma: ...62

Analytical Frameworks for Promoting Health: 63

CHAPTER 8...66

PERSONAL CARE AND ADJUSTMENTS TO DAILY ROUTINES 66

Making Healthy Lifestyle Choices Important: 66

Healthy Eating and Supplement Suggestions: 66

Guidelines for Exercise and Physical Activity 67

Methods for Reducing Stress: 67

Practices for Proper Sleep Hygiene:............68

Taking Care of Your Skin and Sunscreen: ...68

Putting an End to Alcohol and Cigarette Use 69

Overcoming Multiple Chronic Conditions at Once: 69

Methods for Integrative Medicine: 70

Assistive Tools for Wellness: 70

CHAPTER 9 72

RECENT FINDINGS AND PROGRESS IN PITYRIASIS ROSEA RESEARCH 72

New Directions in Scientific Study 72

Research on Biomarkers and Genetics.........73

Immunological Breakthroughs.....................73

Targets for Treatment and Viral Pathways ..74

Experiments in Medicine and Clinical Trials 75

Data Analysis and Epidemiological Surveys 76

Developments in Diagnostic Tools 76

Working Together in Dermatology...............77

Research Initiatives Focused on Patients 78

Looking Ahead: Opportunities and Threats 78

CHAPTER 1 80

PERSONAL NARRATIVES AND VIEWS FROM PATIENTS 80

My Own Story with Pityriasis Rosea 80

Affecting Everyday Life and Interpersonal Connections..................................81

The Path to a Prognosis and Therapy 82

Dealing with Adversity and Building Resilience..................................83

Working to Raise Awareness and Advocacy 84

Recovery Stories That Inspire 85

What I've Learned and What Other People Can Do 86

Community Involvement and Support Groups 86

Patients' Voices Empowered 87

Final Thoughts and Plans for the Future.....88

CHAPTER 1

PITYRIASIS ROSEA: A BRIEF OVERVIEW

Preface and Definition

A self-limiting skin illness known as pityriasis rosea (PR) often affects the trunk, but can also show up on the limbs and neck in the form of oval-shaped, scaly red or pink patches. It typically goes away on its own after a few weeks or months and isn't contagious. Although the precise reason behind PR remains a mystery, it is thought to be associated with viral infections, including HHV-6 and HHV-7. PR is usually diagnosed by observing the patient's symptoms and may not always necessitate medical intervention.

The Past and Its Impact

Gilbert, a French physician, was the first to describe pityriasis rosea in the early 1800s. "Pityriasis" means skin scaling, and "rosea" means the lesions are pinkish-red in color.

Research into PR's causes, symptoms, and management has advanced our understanding of the disease and its therapeutic options.

Research on the Causes and Rates of Pityriasis Rosea

There is little gender bias in the onset of Pityriasis Rosea, which typically strikes people between the ages of 10 and 35. Spring and autumn seem to be the busiest times for it, and it's more prevalent in milder regions. Some areas have a higher reported prevalence of PR than others. Although PR is often thought of as a harmless illness, it has the potential to cause considerable pain and suffering in certain individuals.

Causes and Potential Hazards

Thought to be caused by viral infections, specifically HHV-6 and HHV-7, the precise cause of PR is yet unknown. Stress, hormonal shifts, and a person's genetic makeup are other potential contributors to PR. Some things that can put you at risk include drugs, close contact with people who have **PR**, and recent infections of the upper respiratory tract.

Its Symptoms and Clinical Presentation

One big lesion, known as the "herald patch," is the traditional starting point for pityriasis rosea. Subsequently, smaller lesions spread out in a symmetrical pattern throughout the trunk and, in rare cases, even reach the extremities. The lesions typically have a small number of scales and are oval; they might be red or pink. Lesions may be more visible after vigorous exercise or hot baths, and patients may feel slight itching.

Possible Diagnosis

Some of the symptoms of PR are similar to those of other skin disorders, including eczema, secondary syphilis, medication responses, and tinea corporis (ringworm). Separating PR from these other illnesses and making a definitive diagnosis may need a comprehensive medical history, physical exam, and, in some cases, a skin biopsy.

Techniques for Diagnosis

Clinical manifestations and physical exam results are the mainstays of a Pityriasis Rosea diagnosis. If HHV-6 or HHV-7 DNA is detected, it may be analyzed using viral serology or polymerase chain reaction (PCR), two laboratory techniques. To confirm that the lesions are not caused by anything else, a skin biopsy may be taken.

Concerns and Future Outlook

Typically, PR clears up on its own after 6-8 weeks without any problems. Secondary bacterial infections, post-inflammatory hyperpigmentation (skin darkening), and, extremely infrequently, persistent or recurring PR are problems that may arise. Minimal long-term consequences on skin health contribute to PR's great overall prognosis.

Approaches to Treatment

Symptom alleviation and supportive care are the main goals of treatment for Pityriasis Rosea. If your skin is itchy and inflamed, your doctor may recommend a topical corticosteroid, antihistamine, or emollient. Hot showers, heavy perspiration, and harsh soaps are all things that patients should try to avoid because they could make their symptoms worse. Although the effectiveness of oral antiviral drugs is debatable, they may be considered in cases that are severe or chronic.

Education and Support for Patients

Effective public relations management relies heavily on patient education. It is important to let patients know that their disease is self-limiting, that it will resolve on its own, and that they may manage their symptoms in the meantime. Empowering patients to take charge of their health during PR flare-ups can be achieved by stressing the significance of gentle skin care, avoiding irritants, and seeking medical help for problems.

Pityriasis Rosea is defined, contextualized, epidemiologically studied, etiologically determined, clinically presented, and diagnosed, with potential consequences, treatment alternatives, and patient education topics covered in detail in this comprehensive guide.

CHAPTER 2

SKIN PHYSIOLOGY AND ANATOMY

Skin Structure

The skin is the largest organ in the body and is both intricately and gracefully made. There are three primary layers to it: the dermis, the epidermis, and the hypodermis, or subcutaneous tissue. Protecting us from the elements and keeping us from drying out, the epidermis is the top layer of skin. Melanocytes are located there as well; these are the ones that make the pigment that gives skin its color.

The dermis is below the epidermis and houses the skin's blood vessels, nerves, hair follicles, and perspiration glands. In addition to nourishing the skin, it offers structural support. Fat cells, which insulate and act as an energy reserve, make up the majority of the subcutaneous tissue, which is situated beneath the dermis.

The Skin and Its Functions:

Numerous essential tasks are carried out by the skin. It prevents infections and damage by acting as a barrier against pathogens, pollutants, and UV radiation. In addition to perspiration and the dilatation and constriction of blood vessels, the skin controls core body temperature.

Not only that, but it's a sensitive organ that can pick up on things like pressure, heat, pain, and touch. Another important process for healthy bones is vitamin D production, which occurs when the skin is exposed to sunshine.

The Language of Dermatology:

Various skin disorders, structures, and procedures are described using the extensive vocabulary of dermatology. Some typical terminology includes skin inflammation (dermatitis), redness (erythema), itching (pruritis), and little raised bumps (papules). In dermatology, proper diagnosis and communication rely on familiarity with these words.

Taking Care of Your Skin and Immune System:

Maintaining healthy skin is an immune system priority. An integral part of the skin's immune system, skin-associated lymphoid tissue (SALT) aids in the fight against infections. Langerhans cells, T cells, and other immune cells scour the skin for invaders and destroy them.

In autoimmune diseases like psoriasis and eczema, the immune system attacks healthy skin cells, leading to a variety of skin problems.

How Hormones Affect Skin Disorders:

The condition of one's skin can be affected by hormones including testosterone, estrogen, and cortisol. The increased sebum production that occurs as a result of hormonal changes throughout puberty, for instance, might lead to acne. In a similar vein, dryness, and thinning of the skin might be symptoms of menopausal estrogen swings.

Acne and hirsutism (excessive hair growth) are two skin concerns that can result from hormonal abnormalities, which are observed in disorders such as polycystic ovarian syndrome (PCOS).

Skin Disorders and Heredity:

Many skin problems have strong hereditary components. There is a hereditary component to conditions such as albinism, vitiligo, and hereditary hemochromatosis. Melanoma risk, pigmentation, and skin type are all impacted by hereditary factors.

Accurate diagnosis, treatment, and genetic counseling depend on a thorough understanding of the genetic component of skin problems.

Matters Influencing the Skin from the Environment:

Factors in the environment that can harm the skin are always there. Sunlight's ultraviolet (UV) rays are a leading environmental cause of skin cancer, premature aging, and sunburn. Skin can become dry, irritated, and inflammatory as a result of exposure to chemicals, severe weather, and pollution.

Taking precautions like using sunscreen, being properly hydrated, and staying away from environmental toxins is crucial for keeping skin healthy.

Skin Alterations as a Result of Ageing:

The skin goes through a lot of changes as we get older. Reduced production of collagen and elastin causes a softening and firming of the skin. The skin dries out, gets thinner, and becomes more prone to sagging and wrinkles as we age.

Skin healing is impacted by age-related changes, which make older people more wound-prone and have slower recovery durations. To lessen the severity of these impacts, adopt healthier behaviors and use proper skincare products.

How to Take Care of Your Skin:

To keep skin in good condition, it is necessary to follow good skincare routines. Included in this are routine washes to eliminate oil and grime, moisturizing treatments to avoid dryness, and sun protection to shield from harmful ultraviolet rays. Exfoliation is a great way to get rid of dead skin cells, which in turn increases cell turnover and makes your skin look more beautiful.

It is critical to select skincare products that are suitable for one's skin type and address certain difficulties. Diet, hydration, and stress management are supplementary lifestyle variables that influence skin health.

How Your Diet Affects Your Skin's Condition:

When it comes to skin health, nutrition is king. Proper skin function and repair depend on essential nutrients such as zinc, selenium, and vitamins A, C, E, and D. Antioxidants aid in preventing free radical oxidative damage to skin cells.

Skin health begins on the inside with a well-balanced diet that includes plenty of water, fruits, and vegetables as well as healthy fats. Skin problems including dullness, dryness, and acne can be exacerbated by unhealthy eating habits, lack of water, and too much sweets and alcohol.

CHAPTER 3

HOW PITYRIASIS ROSEA DEVELOPS

How Pityriasis Rosea Develops

Papules that are red and scaly in appearance are the hallmarks of pityriasis rosea (PR), a common skin condition that resolves on its own. Several ideas help us comprehend its etiology, but its exact cause is still a mystery. The exact cause of PR is unknown, however, one popular explanation attributes it to a virus, most likely a human herpesvirus (HHV) like HHV-6 or HHV-7.

The Immunological Processes At Work

According to immunology, PR is linked to a type IV delayed hypersensitivity reaction, which suggests that cytokines and T cells are involved. The characteristic skin lesions seen in PR are thought to be caused by an immunological response that is initiated by a viral infection.

Things That Can Set Off a Virus and How It Can Spread

There is still a lack of clarity regarding the specific viral causes and infection routes in PR. But there's a theory that suggests the virus may enter a latent phase after the first encounter before any symptoms appear. The inflammatory response observed in PR is believed to be influenced by viral replication and dispersion within the skin.

Cytokines and T Cells: Their Function

The pathophysiology of PR is greatly influenced by cytokines and T cells. The skin lesions are invaded by activated T cells, which then secrete pro-inflammatory cytokines like IL-2, IL-6, and TNF-α. It is the reddening and scaling of PR lesions that are a result of these cytokines.

Determinants of Autoimmune Diseases

Although PR is not technically an autoimmune condition, immune-mediated processes play a role in its development. T-cell activation and cytokine release point to an immunological reaction to viral antigens, not an autoimmune attack on host tissues.

The Role of Heredity

While the exact genetic components that contribute to PR remain unknown, there is some evidence that suggests a hereditary propensity. The clustering of instances within families and individual differences in susceptibility raises the possibility of a hereditary component to PR development.

Impacts on the Environment

The frequency and intensity of PR may be affected by environmental variables such as weather, time of year, and geographic region. As an example, PR seems to be more common in temperate regions and at specific seasons, which could indicate that environmental factors have a role.

Factors related to hormones

Some researchers believe that hormonal factors, especially those associated with pregnancy, play a role in the development of PR. Possibly because of hormonal changes impacting immunological responses, some research has shown that the incidence of PR increases during pregnancy.

Changes in Skin Lesions Caused by Pathology

Perivascular lymphocytic infiltration in the dermis, parakeratosis, and epidermal hyperplasia are nonspecific features seen histologically in PR lesions. The skin's reaction to PR, which is inflammatory, is reflected in these alterations.

Reactions Causing Inflammation

The recruitment of immune cells, especially T cells, to the skin lesions characterizes the inflammatory reactions in PR. Activated T cell cytokines cause PR's redness, swelling, and itching by promoting vasodilation, increased vascular permeability, and the migration of inflammatory cells.

Immune responses, viral triggers, environmental factors, genetic and hormonal impacts, environmental factors affecting skin lesions, and inflammatory changes are all important components in understanding the pathophysiology of Pityriasis Rosea. Research on this fascinating skin disorder is ongoing, and although the exact mechanisms are still not fully known, it is providing light on the condition.

CHAPTER 4

FACTORS AND VARIANTS IN CLINICAL PRACTICE

Pityriasis rosea in its traditional form:

The "herald patch" is the initial outward sign of pityriasis rosea (PR). It is usually big, pink, or red, and has a scaly or raised border. The patch can be round or oval in shape. Smaller patches with a similar appearance spread out throughout the body after the first patch has appeared, creating a pattern that looks like a Christmas tree. Typically, the diameter of these secondary patches is only a few millimeters to a few centimeters. While the rash mainly appears on the trunk, it has the potential to extend to other areas such as the legs, arms, and neck.

Unusual and Atypical Variants:

While most people experience PR in its traditional form, there are several uncommon and odd variations. One of these variations is inverted PR, which manifests as a rash in folds of skin like the underarms, groin, or armpits. The development of blisters packed with fluid is a hallmark of vesicular PR, another form of the condition. The lack of a comprehensive evaluation makes diagnosis difficult in cases of other rare variations that manifest with a more extensive or severe rash.

Progression and Clinical Stages

PR usually develops through different phases in the course of its treatment. In the one to two weeks following the appearance of the herald patch, other patches will begin to form. Mild discomfort or itching may be felt by patients at this point. After reaching its height 2–6 weeks later, the rash often fades away over a few weeks to months. As the rash goes away, the skin could look scaly, but scars are usually not left behind.

Skin Lesion Morphology

Round or oval in shape, PR skin lesions can range in color from pink to red, and they often have small scales covering their surface. Lesions can often take on a slightly elevated shape or become ring-shaped when a collarette of scale forms around their margins. You might notice a gradual change in color from red to brown or even grey as the rash goes away.

Patterns of Distribution:

The rash usually shows up on both sides of the body in a symmetrical pattern, which is typical of PR lesions. Atypical variants, in particular, can exhibit distributional variances. The trunk, then the limbs, the neck, and, rarely, the face, are the most typical sites of infection.

Signs & Symptoms, Including Itching:

A common symptom of PR is itching, or pruritus, although the strength of the itching might vary from person to person. While some patients may hardly notice any itching at all, others may find it extremely irritating. Mild exhaustion, headache, and, very infrequently, low-grade fever are some possible signs of PR. In most cases, these systemic symptoms will go away on their own when the rash does.

Differences in Display Based on Gender and Age:

PR is more prevalent in people aged 10–35, while it can happen at any age. The occurrence in females may be slightly higher, although it affects both sexes equally. A more extensive rash or unusual symptoms may be more common in elderly persons and children than in younger adults.

Effects on People's Standard of Living:

Although PR does not pose a life-threatening threat, the itching and concerns about appearance caused by the rash can greatly diminish the quality of life. It could make you feel awkward and self-conscious, especially if the rash is noticeable or hits exposed skin.

Effects on the Mind and Emotions:

Some people may experience psychological and emotional distress as a result of the rash's visibility and the possibility of others misinterpreting it. Patients may feel a range of emotions, including anxiety, embarrassment, and frustration when dealing with symptoms that they find ugly, continuous itching, or recurrent bouts.

Consequences in the Long Run:

Most people with PR can get over it without any lasting effects. After the rash goes away, some individuals may notice a change in their skin tone called post-inflammatory hyperpigmentation or hypopigmentation.

While most people's pigmentation returns to normal within a few months, these changes can last for a while. Although PR can reoccur in extremely rare cases, it usually does not lead to long-term or irreversible skin damage.

CHAPTER 5

ASSESSMENT FOR DIAGNOSIS

Evaluating the Clinical

Synopsis

The characteristic scaly lesions of pityriasis rosea are a feature of this widespread, self-limiting skin illness. It typically begins with a herald patch and progresses to a secondary eruption that is more extensive; it mainly affects young people.

Patient's medical records

An exhaustive medical history must be taken. Some important points are:

- How long the rash lasts and when it starts

The accompanying symptoms, such as itching, fever, and generalized malaise

• Any recent health problems

- All medications taken

- Past skin disorders in the family

Signs • Signs

- **Herald Patch:** A singular, sizable, oval-shaped patch that can be pink or salmon in color and can be seen on the trunk.

A "Christmas tree" pattern of numerous smaller lesions, called a secondary rash, may appear anywhere from a few days to a few weeks following the herald patch. These lesions usually follow Langer's lines of skin tension.

- **Pruritus:** The level of itching can vary, although it is common.

Evaluation of Skin Conditions

Visual Evaluation

- **Herald Patch:** The first lesion, characterised by a delineated scaly border and usually larger than successive ones.

Small, oval spots covered with fine scales, typically found on the trunk and proximal limbs, are called secondary lesions.

How Things Are Distributed

The rash usually doesn't affect the soles of the feet, hands, or cheeks.

The distribution of lesions is often symmetrical.

The Lesions' Development

Before healing, lesions may progress from an erythematous to a hyperpigmented state.

Options for Contemplating a Different Diagnosis

Typical Causes to Dismiss

The presence of ring-like lesions, which may be verified using KOH preparation, is indicative of a fungal infection known as tinea corporis.

Secondary syphilis, which often manifests with systemic symptoms, can also cause a rash that is identical to the first. Serological testing has verified it.

- **Guttate Psoriasis:** Tiny, pimple-like lesions that are coated in skin flake and typically appear after a streptococcal infection.

Eczema, also known as atopic dermatitis, is a chronic skin illness characterized by recurrent episodes and a unique pattern of occurrence.

Less Common Illnesses

Drug Eruptions: The patient's history confirms the presence of a rash that occurs after taking medicine.

It is common for children to experience viral exanthems, which are associated with systemic symptoms.

Procedures and Tests for Diagnosis

• Peeling Off Dead Skin

It is possible to use a potassium hydroxide (KOH) solution on skin scrapings to detect and eliminate fungal diseases, such as tinea corporis.

Serological Evaluations

To rule out secondary syphilis, you can undergo testing with Rapid Plasma Reagin (RPR) or the Venereal Disease Research Laboratory (VDRL).

Testing for Bugs

- In cases where allergies may have been present in the past, to rule out the possibility of allergic contact dermatitis.

Results from Histopathology

Use Cases for Biopsies

Although not usually necessary, it may be done in cases where the diagnosis is not obvious or when unusual symptoms manifest.

Common Discoveries

-Slight thickening of the epidermis, also known as mild hyperkeratosis

- Maintaining cell nuclei in the outermost layer of the skin (parakeratosis)

- Epidermal intercellular edema, also known as focal spongiosis

-The dermis shows signs of perivascular lymphocytic infiltration

Studies Conducted in a Lab

Standard Evaluations

Usually isn't required in most circumstances.

Particular Evaluations

- Although not commonly done, viral cultures or polymerase chain reaction (PCR) may be included in the investigation of possible infectious causes.

** Imaging Research

Imaging's Function

Since pityriasis rosea is best diagnosed by a careful skin examination, imaging investigations are usually not utilized for this purpose.

Diagnosis Requirements

Important Requirements

- A herald patch is present.

- A second rash that develops after Langer's lines

- A self-contained process that resolves on its own

Minor Requirements

- Faint initial symptoms (such as lethargy or a headache)

The lack of major systemic symptoms

Verification"

The manifestation and development of the rash are the most important clinical features in making a diagnosis.

Issues with Diagnosis

Unusual Displays

- Other types of pityriasis rosea include vesicular, purpuric, and inverse pityriasis rosea, which manifests as lesions on the limbs instead of the trunk.

Possible Diagnosis

It can be more challenging to diagnose if symptoms are similar to those of other dermatoses.

Delays in Diagnosis

It is possible to overtreat a patient due to a false diagnosis of a fungal infection or another dermatosis.

A Critical Aspect of Prompt Identification

Assuring the Patient

-Assuring the patient of the correct diagnosis can assist ease their concerns over the rash's cause.

The Right Way to Manage

- Steer clear of therapies that aren't essential and could do more harm than good (such as antibiotics and antifungals, for example).

Keeping Tabs and Following Up

The anticipated progression and the necessity of symptomatic medication (such as antihistamines for itching) can be identified and advised upon.

Implications for Public Health

- Realising that pityriasis rosea does not transmit very well from person to person, which alleviates unnecessary anxiety about the disease's potential spread.

Pityriasis rosea can be better managed, patients can feel more at ease, and unneeded therapies can be avoided with a prompt and precise diagnosis. Healthcare personnel must be well-versed in the clinical features and differential diagnosis to provide the best possible care.

CHAPTER 6

METHODS FOR CONTROL AND REHABILITATION

A Primer on Management Theory and Practice

1. **Confirmation of Diagnosis:** Verification of a correct diagnosis using a thorough clinical examination and, if necessary, a skin biopsy.

2. Assure them that Pityriasis Rosea will go away on its own and educate them on the condition's benign course.

3. **Avoid Triggers:** Advise patients to stay out of direct sunlight and away from harsh skincare products, since these can be triggers.

4. Assist with symptoms like pruritus (itching) and pain by implementing strategies to alleviate them.

Counseling and Education for Patients

1. **Condition Overview:** Affirm that Pityriasis Rosea is harmless and will go away on its own to put patients at ease.

2. **Illness Progression** Outline the normal sequence in which a rash could develop, worsen, and eventually go away.

3. **Symptom Management:** Make sure patients know how to deal with itching and pain by providing them with the right information.

4. To keep tabs on progress and provide comfort, it's crucial to schedule follow-up appointments.

Pharmaceutical Approaches

1. Oral antihistamines might be prescribed to alleviate pruritus symptoms.

2. For intense or localized irritation, you may want to look into using topical steroids, especially those with a lower potency.

3. If the condition is severe or if there are noticeable systemic symptoms, the patient may be prescribed oral steroids.

4. **Antiviral Agents:** When a viral cause is recognized or suspected, these agents may be used.

Treatments Applied Topically

1. To alleviate dry, itchy skin, use an emollient or moisturizer.

2. **Calamine Lotion:** Apply calamine lotion to the affected area to alleviate itching and chill down.

3. Consider using a topical antihistamine for localized pruritus; however, there is less data to support this.

Systemic therapies

1. For moderate to severe pruritus that topical treatments are unable to control, consider using oral antihistamines.

2. In extreme circumstances or if systemic symptoms manifest, systemic steroids may be considered.

3. Controversial, but worth considering in some cases, is antiviral therapy.

Non-Conventional and Allied Medical Practices

1. There is a paucity of scientific evidence for herbal remedies, therefore patients should be warned about possible interactions.

2. A lack of data has led to anecdotal claims suggesting that acupuncture may help alleviate symptoms.

3. Homoeopathic remedies are controversial, thus it's best to advise people to talk to their doctors before using them.

Managing Itching

1. To alleviate itching, try using cool compresses or taking a cool bath.

2. **Avoid Irritants:** Advise patients to stay away from things that can make their itching worse, such as hot baths, harsh soaps, and tight clothing.

3. To alleviate itching and other symptoms of pruritus, you can use antihistamines, either topically or orally.

Complication Prevention

1. **Sun Protection:** Instruct patients to wear protective clothing and use sunblock to avoid further sunburn.

2. To avoid skin irritation and subsequent infections, it is important to practice gentle skincare.

3. **Avoidance of Allergens:** To minimize flare-ups, advise patients to avoid recognized triggers.

Care Maintenance

1. Make sure to schedule follow-up visits to track the progress of the rash and evaluate how well symptoms are being managed.

2. **Reassurance:** Reassure the patient repeatedly that Pityriasis Rosea is harmless and that the condition will eventually go away.

3. The patient's reaction and the presence or absence of new problems should inform any necessary adjustments to the treatment plan.

Factors that Predict Outcome

1. **Age:** On the whole, younger people tend to have a better prognosis than older adults.

2. **Overall Health:** Patients who are in generally good health tend to recover more quickly.

3. In most cases, complications-free recovery takes longer for patients experiencing severe

itching or systemic symptoms, however, this is not always the case.

This all-encompassing method addresses several facets of Pityriasis Rosea management and treatment, with an emphasis on educating patients, alleviating symptoms, preventing complications, and providing proper follow-up care.

CHAPTER 7

PSYCHOSOCIAL EFFECTS AND METHODS OF COPING

How Pityriasis Rosea Affects the Mind:

The mental impacts of pityriasis rosea can differ from person to person. Some people may feel minor discomfort from the apparent skin issue, while others may have a far more difficult time managing the symptoms. Feelings of shame, nervousness, despair, and annoyance are typical mental side effects. Comprehensive care for persons with pityriasis rosea requires an understanding of these consequences.

Effects on Confidence and Perception of One's Body:

When the rash from pityriasis rosea is noticeable or shows up in public places, it can hurt self-esteem and body image. A person's unfavorable view of their physical attractiveness could stem from feelings of self-consciousness. The promotion of a healthy self-image and mental wellness depends on addressing these problems through supportive treatments.

Methods for Coping and Resources for Help:

When it comes to dealing with the psychological and social effects of pityriasis rosea, effective coping mechanisms are crucial. It might be helpful to encourage patients to do things that make them feel good about themselves, such stay well, relax often, and reach out to friends and family for support. In times of difficulty, support networks such as family, friends, and support groups are there to lend an ear and lend emotional support.

Things to Think About for Your Mental Health:

Anxiety, despair, and heightened stress levels are among the mental health issues that pityriasis rosea patients may face. To address these factors, healthcare providers must conduct thorough evaluations and implement individualized therapies. Patients coping with the mental and physical components of their ailment can benefit from interdisciplinary teams that include mental health experts.

Psychotherapy and Counselling:

The psychological effects of pityriasis rosea can be better managed with the help of counseling and psychotherapy. Individuals can enhance their well-being, build coping mechanisms, and combat negative thought patterns through the use of mindfulness-based practices, supportive counseling, and cognitive-behavioral therapy (CBT). Personalizing therapeutic approaches to meet the unique needs of each patient increases their chances of success and fosters resilience.

Family and social support play an important role:

When dealing with adversity, having the support of loved ones and friends is essential. Support networks can be strengthened by family education about pityriasis rosea, encouragement of open communication, and provision of practical aid. People with the disease can benefit emotionally and socially from reduced isolation and increased opportunities to participate in social activities.

Programmes for Raising Awareness and Education:

As part of psychosocial assistance, it is vital to educate people about pityriasis rosea and raise awareness of the condition. Dispelling falsehoods, reducing stigma, and promoting understanding can be achieved through educational programs targeted at patients, carers, and the community. Providing people with up-to-date information allows them to take charge of their health and embrace their condition.

Promoting Patients' Legal Rights:

Promoting patient access to high-quality care and fighting for patients' rights are two important goals of advocacy work. Better healthcare coverage, more money for research, and more support services are all possible outcomes of collaborative efforts between patient advocacy groups, healthcare organizations, and lawmakers. Overall patient outcomes are improved and advocacy efforts are bolstered when patients are empowered to express their demands.

Confronting Misconceptions and Stigma:

To break down social barriers and promote inclusivity, it is essential to address the stigma and myths surrounding pityriasis rosea. To combat prejudice and promote understanding and tolerance, we need more educational opportunities, more public awareness campaigns, and more community involvement programs. The health of people afflicted by the illness can be improved by making their environment more accepting and less judgmental.

Analytical Frameworks for Promoting Health:

By bringing together one's mental, emotional, and social health, integrative methods take a more complete picture of wellness. Pityriasis rosea patients can benefit from a healthier lifestyle by including stress reduction techniques, a balanced diet, frequent physical activity, and complementary medicine in their routine. Individualized, all-encompassing care is possible when healthcare providers from different fields work together.

Psychological assistance, education, advocacy, and integrative solutions are all necessary to address the psychosocial burden of pityriasis rosea. Healthcare practitioners can help patients with pityriasis rosea enhance their quality of life, resilience, and empowerment by acknowledging and addressing the social and emotional elements of the condition.

CHAPTER 8

PERSONAL CARE AND ADJUSTMENTS TO DAILY ROUTINES

Making Healthy Lifestyle Choices Important:

Effective management of pityriasis rosea requires a commitment to a healthy lifestyle. Making healthy choices can improve your health in general, strengthen your immune system, and maybe alleviate some of your symptoms. The skin and the body's ability to mend itself can both benefit from regular exercise and a balanced diet.

Healthy Eating and Supplement Suggestions:

Essential elements for skin health and immunological function can be found in a balanced diet that is rich in fruits, vegetables, lean meats, and whole grains. Vitamins A, C, and E are antioxidants that may aid in the fight against inflammation and the promotion of skin healing. The skin and general health can both benefit from a diet low in sugar, processed foods, and bad fats.

Guidelines for Exercise and Physical Activity

Engaging in regular physical activity has numerous health benefits, including enhanced circulation, improved immunological function, reduced stress, and improved general well-being. It may be helpful to participate in moderate-intensity exercises like swimming, brisk walking, or yoga. To keep the skin from becoming irritated, though, try not to perspire too heavily or rub the affected regions too vigorously.

Methods for Reducing Stress:

Feelings of stress might make pityriasis rosea worse. One way to lower stress levels is to practice stress management strategies like deep breathing, yoga, meditation, or participating in hobbies. Making time for yourself and reaching out to people you care about, like family or a counselor, can also help.

Practices for Proper Sleep Hygiene:

The immune system and general well-being depend on getting a good night's sleep. To enhance the quality of your sleep, it is recommended that you stick to a regular sleep schedule, develop a soothing routine before bed, and make sure your bedroom is dark, quiet, and has comfy bedding. To help you get a better night's rest, try cutting back on screen time in the hours leading up to bedtime and staying away from stimulants like caffeine.

Taking Care of Your Skin and Sunscreen:

Because ultraviolet radiation can exacerbate skin disorders like pityriasis rosea, it is essential to protect the skin from the sun as much as possible. Always wear protective clothes, use a broad-spectrum sunscreen with an SPF of 30 or greater, and look for shade when the sun is at its strongest. To keep your skin healthy, use gentle skincare products like moisturizers and cleansers.

Putting an End to Alcohol and Cigarette Use

Impaired immune function and worsening skin problems can be caused by smoking and excessive alcohol usage. Better skin health, including less inflammation and faster healing, can be yours when you kick the habit of smoking and cut back on alcohol.

Overcoming Multiple Chronic Conditions at Once:

Efficient management of underlying chronic illnesses is crucial for those with diabetes or autoimmune disorders. To make sure all of your health problems are being well-managed, it's important to listen to your doctor, take your medicine exactly as prescribed, and keep up with your checkups.

Methods for Integrative Medicine:

Acupuncture, herbal supplements, and aromatherapy are examples of complementary therapies that some people may find useful for symptom management and general health support. But if you're already on medicine, it's really important to talk to your doctor before starting anything new.

Assistive Tools for Wellness:

People living with pityriasis rosea can become more self-reliant when they have access to credible self-care resources like support groups, educational materials, and trustworthy websites. Additionally, dermatologists, healthcare practitioners, and support groups can all provide individualized advice and assistance.

CHAPTER 9

RECENT FINDINGS AND PROGRESS IN PITYRIASIS ROSEA RESEARCH

New Directions in Scientific Study

A common skin condition known as Pityriasis Rosea (PR) is marked by a characteristic rash. The current wave of studies is aiming to better understand the processes at work, develop more accurate diagnostic tools, and investigate potential new treatments. To further understand the cause of PR, researchers are making use of cutting-edge technologies including genomics, proteomics, and bioinformatics. Human herpesvirus (HHV)-6 and HHV-7, in particular, are being studied more closely as possible causes. Additionally, there has been an uptick in the use of interdisciplinary research methods; for example, geneticists, dermatologists, and immunologists have all worked together to improve our knowledge of PR.

Research on Biomarkers and Genetics

Discovering possible genetic components that contribute to PR is the goal of genetic investigations. Scientists are using GWAS, or genome-wide association studies, to look for disease-related genetic variations. Research into biomarkers is also on the rise, with the hope of identifying particular biological indicators that can facilitate early diagnosis and individualized treatment. Some examples of biomarkers are immune cell signatures, gene expression profiles, and certain proteins. In addition to assisting with early detection, identifying genetic predispositions and biomarkers can aid in the development of personalized treatment plans.

Immunological Breakthroughs

An important player in PR's pathophysiology is the immune system. The role of adaptive and innate immune responses in PR development has recently been brought to light by research. Evidence of an immunological-mediated component has been found in studies of PR patients, who have higher levels of certain cytokines and immune cells. To learn more about the factors that cause PR to start and worsen, researchers are looking at the intricate web of relationships between the immune system and viral infections. These findings have the potential to pave the way for novel immunomodulatory therapies that target immunological dysregulation in patients with PR.

Targets for Treatment and Viral Pathways

A major function for viral infections, especially HHV-6 and HHV-7, is thought to be in PR. Scientists are currently trying to figure out which viral pathways cause the sickness. New therapeutic targets may be discovered by elucidating the mechanisms by which these viruses bind to host cells and initiate the immune response. Aiming to suppress viral replication and alleviate symptoms, antiviral treatments are being investigated as a potential therapy option. Better patient outcomes may be possible with the creation of targeted antiviral medications, which could be made possible by studying the molecular underpinnings of viral infections.

Experiments in Medicine and Clinical Trials

To ensure the effectiveness and safety of new PR treatments, clinical trials are necessary. Experiments in this category examine both new pharmacological substances and the off-label uses of current pharmaceuticals. Various experimental treatments are presently undergoing clinical trials, including biologics, immunological modulators, and antiviral medicines. Potential non-pharmacological therapies, such as phototherapy, are also being investigated by researchers. To develop evidence-based standards for PR management, the outcomes of these experiments are vital.

Data Analysis and Epidemiological Surveys

To further understand PR's demographic characteristics, incidence, and prevalence, epidemiological surveys are helpful. Age, sex, region, and seasonal changes are some of the risk factors that can be identified by data analysis of these surveys. Public health initiatives to increase awareness and better early identification can be devised by knowing the epidemiology of PR. To further understand the role of environmental and genetic variables in PR, large-scale epidemiological research is invaluable.

Developments in Diagnostic Tools

Diagnostic technology advancements are making PR diagnosis faster and more accurate. The use of dermoscopy, a non-invasive imaging method, to distinguish PR from other comparable skin disorders is on the rise. To detect viral DNA and identify genetic markers, molecular diagnostic methods including next-generation sequencing (NGS) and polymerase chain reaction (PCR) are being used. Accurate diagnosis is the first step in developing effective treatment programs, and these technologies make that possible.

Working Together in Dermatology

To make progress in PR research and treatment, dermatologists, researchers, and other healthcare experts must work together. To share information, do thorough studies, and develop new treatments, interdisciplinary teams are collaborating. Collaborations also include relationships between pharmaceutical corporations, research organizations, and academic institutions. Great strides are made in the sector as a result of these partnerships since they allow for the sharing of data, knowledge, and resources.

Research Initiatives Focused on Patients

Research efforts that put patients' needs and experiences first are known as patient-centered research initiatives. To better understand how PR affects patients' quality of life, these programs encourage them to take part in clinical experiments, questionnaires, and focus groups. Researchers can better address the unique concerns and desires of PR patients by gaining an understanding of patient perspectives. When it comes to getting the word out about the ailment and funding research, patient advocacy groups are also vital.

Looking Ahead: Opportunities and Threats

Combining state-of-the-art methods with fresh ideas is where public relations research is headed. Future studies combining genomic and proteomic data with cutting-edge imaging methods should shed light on the causes and mechanisms of PR.

Still, there are obstacles to overcome, such as increasing the size and diversity of research populations, standardizing diagnostic criteria, and creating effective medicines with little side effects. Sustained financing, worldwide collaboration, and a dedication to patient-centered research are necessary to address these difficulties.

Finally, researchers are making great achievements in the field of Pityriasis Rosea. Researchers hope that by delving further into this illness, they will be able to develop better diagnostic tools and treatments.

CHAPTER 10

PERSONAL NARRATIVES AND VIEWS FROM PATIENTS

My Own Story with Pityriasis Rosea

Getting to Know Pityriasis Rosea

The characteristic rash of pityriasis rosea is a manifestation of this prevalent skin ailment. A single huge pink oval spot, or "herald patch," is the usual beginning point, with subsequent smaller patches appearing all over the body. Even while it's not infectious and often goes away after six to eight weeks, the pain and suffering it causes can be substantial.

Stories from Patients

A lot of people who have pityriasis rosea say it came on quickly and without warning. As an example, Sarah, a teacher in her twenties, recalls waking up one morning with what she initially believed to be a minor allergic response. Worry and bewilderment ensued as her skin became covered in red, scaly spots within days.

A college student named James remembers getting pityriasis rosea while studying for exams. He had to visit a dermatologist to get the proper diagnosis after it was first thought to be eczema. His experience shows how important it is to consult a doctor when you notice any changes to your skin.

Affecting Everyday Life and Interpersonal Connections

Everyday Obstacles

Pityriasis rosea can make it hard to sleep and do everyday things because of how itchy it is. For example, a young mother named Emma had a hard time taking care of her newborn since she was itchy all the time. Feeling self-conscious and hesitant to join in on social events were additional outcomes of the visible rash.

* Connections

Because of the emotional toll it takes, the disease can put a strain on relationships. Isolation may set in because loved ones don't comprehend the full extent of the effect. It was difficult for David to explain his illness to his coworkers and friends. People would ask him awkward questions and make assumptions about his health because the rash was so obvious.

The Path to a Prognosis and Therapy

How to Perform a Diagnosis

Several trips to the doctor are usually necessary to get a proper diagnosis. Many patients, like Laura, may first undergo therapy for other issues, like allergies or fungal infections. Dermatologists typically correctly diagnose pityriasis rosea by reviewing the patient's medical history and doing a physical examination.

Approaches to Treatment

Despite the lack of a cure, pityriasis rosea can be effectively treated with a variety of methods. Itching and inflammation can be effectively managed with over-the-counter antihistamines and topical corticosteroids. The use of ultraviolet radiation in phototherapy helped some patients, like Mark.

Dealing with Adversity and Building Resilience

Methods for Successfully Coping

As a means of dealing with their illness, patients find various ways of coping. Lotions that hydrate the skin, oatmeal baths, and loose clothing can all help with physical comfort. As previously stated, Emma discovered that practicing mindfulness and meditation helped her deal with the emotional and mental toll that her condition took on her.

Creating a Strong Foundation

Being resilient means you know that pityriasis rosea is just a transient, harmless condition. Important roles are played by loved ones, friends, and medical experts. It could be comforting and empowering to talk to people who have been through the same things you have.

Working to Raise Awareness and Advocacy

Getting the Word Out

For early diagnosis and stigma reduction, it is vital to raise knowledge of pityriasis rosea. Blogging, social media, and support group sharing of personal stories is a common tactic in advocacy activities. Groups and individuals are making an effort to raise awareness of the illness among healthcare providers and the general public.

The Part Played by Medical Professionals

As advocates, healthcare personnel should educate themselves on the condition and its treatment choices, as well as keep up with the newest research in the field. A patient's experience and outlook can be greatly enhanced via compassionate communication.

Recovery Stories That Inspire

Overcoming Obstacles

Pityriasis rosea can be a real obstacle, yet many people have overcome it. For instance, Sophia used her time spent dealing with a chronic skin issue to write a book that others can use as a guide.

Determining Your Goals

Just like Alex, some patients can help others by sharing their stories. A feeling of community and unity has been fostered by Alex's local support group, where members offer emotional support and share suggestions.

What I've Learned and What Other People Can Do

Main Points

Patience and self-care are frequently emphasised by patients. Reducing anxiousness is possible when you know that pityriasis rosea goes away on its own. Sarah encourages people to listen to their dermatologists and not scratch to avoid further infections.

Tips for First-Time Patients

It is critical for people who have just received a diagnosis to find trustworthy resources and make connections with individuals who understand what they are going through. For those in need of insight and emotional support, many suggest getting involved in internet forums or finding a local support group.

Community Involvement and Support Groups

Perks of Having a Support System

People can feel comfortable opening out and receiving guidance in support groups. In addition to offering practical advice for symptom management, they also offer emotional support. People with first-hand knowledge of Pityriasis rosea typically spearhead these support groups, which can be located both online and in local areas.

Engaging with the Community

One way to make people feel more at home is to get them involved in community events and awareness campaigns. Help raise awareness and funds for research by taking part in walks, fundraisers, or educational programs.

Patients' Voices Empowered

Narrative Sharing

Patients might find strength and healing by opening up about their experiences. Sharing one's story can help break down barriers, lessen prejudice, and offer solace to individuals going through tough times.

Forums for Opinions

Community support and advocacy can be strengthened by establishing online spaces where patients can share their stories, including social media groups, podcasts, or blogs. Newly diagnosed patients might also find helpful information and comfort on these platforms.

Final Thoughts and Plans for the Future

Research and awareness must be ongoing.

To advance our understanding of pityriasis rosea and its treatment possibilities, further research is necessary. Better patient outcomes and earlier diagnoses are possible results of heightened awareness.

Looking on the Bright Side

Despite how difficult pityriasis rosea can be, keep in mind that it is only a transient and treatable ailment. Full and active lives are within reach for patients with the correct support systems, treatments, and self-care practices. Everyone impacted by this condition can take heart in the fact that patients, healthcare providers, and activists are working together to make a difference.

www.ingramcontent.com/pod-product-compliance
Lightning Source LLC
Chambersburg PA
CBHW061252250726
48653CB00002B/621